INTERMITTENT FASTING PLANNER & HEALTH GUIDE

lose weight fast between 0.8% - 3.0% of
baseline body weight within 12 weeks

Tracy Webb

CONTENTS

INTRODUCTION

O ver time, people have devised many ways to lose weight. These diets often become fads and could be detrimental to one's health. Fasting is generally considered a way to lose weight, but if done right, intermittent fasting can be of great benefit to your health, and the prevalence of this type of fasting has greatly increased in the past few years (Barnosky, Hoddy, Unterman, & Varady 2014).

We will try to show you the pros and the cons of fasting. The idea is to show you how some people can benefit from it. Diet may affect the body's insulin levels, human growth hormone, affect the body's gene expression and increase cell repair.

Most people go on a diet to lose weight, and intermittent fasting is one of many methods. The most important thing is the struggle between belly fat and the battle to get rid of it. The key is to eat the right food, because if you eat high-calorie food after fasting, it will be useless. This is one of the reasons why fasting might not work for some (Gunnars 2016).

As I said at the beginning, it's all about doing it right and deciding why you want to do it. Combine fasting with the right diet, for example, you may find that it is an effective way to lose weight. However, as we have already mentioned, many health benefits can be obtained from it.

It is also important to understand that there are different ways to fast intermittently. This has to do with how you divide your meal times and your fasting periods. An example is the "Eat stop Eat" method, which requires that you should fast for twenty-four hours at least once a week. You can also be fast twice a week. Another example is the 16:8 fasting diet, which indicates that you fast for 14-16 hours a day and that you have a daily eating time of 8-10 hours (Gunnars 2020).

This booklet will give you insight and an overview of intermittent fasting as a guide to health and weight loss. One of the most important aspects of any diet is to consult your doctor, especially if you have any underlying illnesses or even just for a peace of mind.

For any of these methods to work, it is vital that you make this a part of your normal schedule. Simply put, you need to normalize it and integrate it into your lifestyle. The latter is especially true for intermittent fasting as a religious activity. However, this idea is a personal choice, and it is possible that you do this only for a limited time.

CHAPTER 1: THE
DIFFERENT TYPES OF
INTERMITTENT FASTING

T he intermittent fasting strategy is not a diet, but a pattern of eating. It is a cycle of eating that one can turn into a habit. This eating pattern does not include a particular diet. This means that you do not need to eat certain types of food, but only needs to eat different foods than before, that is, change the time of eating (Gunnars 2017). Hence, you can use an intermittent fasting strategy in the following ways:

Method 16/8 Or Leangains Protocol

This method is especially popular among fitness enthusiasts.However, you can also use it, but remember to consult a doctor. The Leangains protocol is also geared at muscle gain. Succeeding this protocol would mean a more prescribed diet, though (Owings). For an ordinary person, though, it is easy to follow, as you can decide what you would like to eat during the window the method allows for.

An example of this method is that you fast for 14-16 hours a day and eat within a period of 8-10 hours. The idea is that, for example, you will stop eating before 8pm. Then, your fast will start and continue until 12 o'clock in the afternoon until you start your first meal. A snack would mean a break in your fast. You do this every day:

METHOD 16/8	
One Day	
4 am 8 am	Your Fasting period from Midnight
12 pm	Your first meal of the day
8 pm	Your last meal of the day
8 pm Midnight	Your fast starts

Table 1: Extracted from Gunner 2020

Your mealtime is between your first meal and your last meal. You can eat as many meals as you like (Gunnars 2020). However, you have to keep in mind your reason for doing this. That would then mean you have to ensure that you do not overeat or eat unhealthy foods

The 5:2 Method

In this method, you usually have a normal diet for 5 out of the 7 days of the week, but restrict your diet on the other two days. This idea is not a complete fast, because you still have to eat, but if you are a female, you will only eat two small meals, each with 250 calories, and if you are a male, 300 calories per meal for the remaining two days. For men, this would be equal to 600 calories, for women, it would be equal to 500 calories. However, these figures are only suggestive (Gunnars 2020).

5:2 METHOD						
Day 1	Day 2	Day 3	Day 4	Day 5	Day 6	Day 7
Eat Nor-mally	Calories to eat: Male: 600 Female: 500	Eat Nor-mally	Eat Nor-mally	Calories to eat: Male: 600 Female: 500	Eat Nor-mally	Eat Nor-mally

Table 2: Extracted from Gunner 2020

The 'Eat Stop Eat' Method

It is similar to the 5:2 method, the difference is that you can completely fast for 2 days in 7 days. You usually eat on 5 of the 7 days, and then fast for 24 hours during those two days.

The 'Eat Stop Eat' Method						
Day 1	Day 2	Day 3	Day 4	Day 5	Day 6	Day 7
Eat Normally	Fast for 24 hours	Eat Normally	Eat Normally	Fast for 24 hours	Eat Normally	Eat Normally

Table 3: Extracted from Gunner 2020

Fasting On Alternate Days

This method of intermittent fasting is to alternate fasting or low-calorie meals.For example, you can fast completely on three days of the week (i.e., every other day) and then eat some calorie food. You can also alternate it from one week to the other as well.

Fasting on Alternate Days						
Day 1	Day 2	Day 3	Day 4	Day 5	Day 6	Day 7
Eat Nor-mally	Fast for 24 hours Or Eat limite d Cal-ories	Eat Nor-mally	Fast for 24 hours Or Eat limite d Cal-ories	Eat Nor-mally	Fast for 24 hours Or Eat limite d Cal-ories	Eat Nor-mally

Table 4: Extracted from Gunner 2020

The Warrior Diet

The difference with the Warrior diet is that it allows you to fast for a whole day and then eat a lot of food at night (Gunnars 2020).

It is called the "Warrior Diet" because the ancient warriors did not eat all day, but only had a big meal at night. People who use this method will eat some healthy snacks, such as dairy products, with a small amount of fruits and vegetables in between (Kubala 2018).

THE WARRIOR DIET							
	Day 1	Day 2	Day 3	Day 4	Day 5	Day 6	Day 7
20 hours of fasting	Eat snacks, such as a small portion of fruits and vegetables	Eat snacks, such as a small portion of fruits and vegetables	Eat snacks, such as a small portion of fruits and vegetables	Eat snacks, such as a small portion of fruits and vegetables	Eat snacks, such as a small portion of fruits and vegetables	Eat snacks, such as a small portion of fruits and vegetables	Eat snacks, such as a small portion of fruits and vegetables
Within a 4-hour window	Eat one large meal	Eat one large meal	Eat one large meal	Eat one large meal	Eat one large meal	Eat one large meal	Eat one large meal

Table 5: Extracted from Gunner 2020

Randomly Omitting Meals

This is a much easier route to go as you can decide whenever you feel like skipping a meal. For example, if you get up in the morning, you can decide whether you are going to have breakfast or not. This could be once every week or more. You could also decide which day you are going to skip dinner or not. This idea too can be once a week, or even more. The idea is to randomly decide when you want to skip a meal.

RANDOMLY OMITTING MEALS							
	Day 1	Day 2	Day 3	Day 4	Day 5	Day 6	Day 7
Breakfast	Eat	Eat	No Breakfast	Eat	Eat	Eat	Eat
Lunch	Eat	Eat	Eat	Eat	Eat	Eat	Eat
Dinner	Eat	Eat	Eat	Eat	No Dinner	Eat	Eat

Table 6: Extracted from Gunner 2020

It is recommended that you do not perform any of these fasting methods without medical supervision. If you can, you should involve a health practitioner in the decisions you make as far as intermittent fasting is concerned. The reason you choose to do this is that, you want to live a healthier life, so you don't want to harm your body in any way.

CHAPTER 2: THE
PROS AND CONS OF
INTERMITTENT FASTING

A ll diets, including intermittent fasting, have their advantages and disadvantages. The intermittent fast is not always beneficial to some, but it could be helpful if used correctly. Therefore, it is important to understand your body and what works for you. Here are some pros and cons for you to consider:

The Pros Of Intermittent Fasting

Intermittent fasting improves your blood sugar levels

As a direct health benefit, intermittent fasting improves the insulin levels in your body. It can prevent Type 2 diabetes. This way of fasting, therefore, helps the body control its sugar levels (Barnosky, Hoddy, Unterman, & Varady 2014). The purpose of insulin in the body is to regulate blood sugar levels. If this is not controlled it can lead to diabetes or weight gain. By making intermittent fasting a habit, you are able to lower blood sugar levels. This means that your insulin will drop as well. This will promote fat burning and weight loss (The Mayo Clinic Staff 2019).

Intermittent fasting increases your growth hormones and prepares your cells

1. Increase in Growth Hormones

The growth hormones in the body ensure that your body has healthy muscles and build fat around the body. Healthy fat is necessary to protect parts of the body, but belly fat has a habit of getting out of hand. The hormones are also valuable to maintain the balance between the densities of the lipoproteins in your cholesterol levels. It further maintains bone density. What's more, your growth hormone is necessary for your brain function.

Intermittent fasting has the ability to increase the blood levels of your growth hormone. This is where higher levels of hormones can burn fat and build more muscle (Gunnars 2016).

2. Reparation at Cellular Level

Intermittent fasting is good for cell repair, because the body is at rest, so it also has the opportunity to remove toxins and other waste (Gunnars 2016).

Intermittent Fasting helps you with weight loss and loss of belly fat

The discussion here touched on intermittent fasting as a way to lose weight. This idea is also an important factor in reducing belly fat. Losing weight and reducing belly fat are some of the reasons why most people choose to fast. Studies have shown that fasting can increase your metabolism by 3.6-14%, and can help you burn more calories (Gunnars, 2016). Most importantly, intermittent fasting helps reduce calories and, hence, archived to weight loss (Barnosky, Hoddy, Unterman, & Varady 2014)

Other ways in which Intermittent Fasting can benefit you

Intermittent fasting can be of benefit in the long term. You might be able to live a longer life. We have mentioned how this kind of fasting can help your body at the cellular level by the renewal of cells. The renewal of cells is related to longevity (Goodrick, Ingram, Reynolds, Freeman, & Cider 1983),

The Cons Of Intermittent Fasting

The benefits of intermittent fasting can outweigh the cons. Some of the cons of this type of fasting are that (Harvard Health):

1. Most people do not persist with the process. As Harvard Health states, there is a 38% dropout rate, which inadvertently leads to failure in weight loss. Because it is a fasting regime, people are likely to eat more after a 14-16 hour fast and, thus, overeat.

2. The difficulty for most people trying out fasting is that they might not be backing it up with a healthy eating plan. As I said before, you have to do it the right way for it to work.

3. Some restaurants will provide some ready-made food packaging intermittently, but the downside is that it may be too expensive in the long run.

4. Even if there is evidence that intermittent fasting can help prevent cancer and strengthen the body, there is no guarantee that it is effective. Therefore, most people only consider it as a weight loss plan.

CHAPTER 3: THE HEALTH BENEFITS OF INTERMITTENT FASTING

Although as highlighted the pros and cons of intermittent fasting, it is worth seeing what benefits it has for health. Some of the influences of fasting can have a direct effect on the major organs of the body. Here are some examples:

1. The effect of Intermittent Fasting on the Liver
Intermittent fasting allows the body to slowly consume the glucose that is stored in the liver. It takes about 10 to 12 hours to do so. When this happens, the energy in the liver is used up and the body is forced to fat-burning to generate energy (Thompson 2019).

2. The effect of Intermittent Fasting on Blood Pressure
According to Lawler et al, intermittent fasting can lower high blood pressure in the short run. This means that it only lasts while the person is on the regime. As soon as stop the eating pattern, the blood levels would return to normal. Studies have shown that it is especially the top number of the blood pressure measurement – that is, the systolic blood pressure. Normal and healthy blood pressure can prevent kidney disease, strokes, and heart disease (Lawler et al).

3. The effect of Intermittent Fasting on the Heart
   i.   In conjunction with lowering the blood pressure, intermittent fasting can also protect your heart against any cardiovascular diseases. The effect of

intermittent fasting has on the liver and so metabolism, helps lower triglyceride levels as well as blood sugar levels that have a direct influence on the health of the heart (Lawler et a).

ii. A secondary aspect that would affect the heart is that intermittent fasting can also lower cholesterol.

4. The effect of Intermittent Fasting on Most Parts of the Body Inflammation can occur in a number of different parts of the body. Studies have shown that reducing calorie intake during intermittent fasting can reduce inflammation. The study specifically pointed out the fasting system of Muslims. It was pointed out that when the subjects fasted, the inflammation index was lower (Lawler et al).

CHAPTER 4: THE SIDE EFFECTS AND SOLUTIONS OF INTERMITTENT FASTING

E ven though some disadvantages are mentioned in Chapter 2, please alllow me to explain the side effects of intermittent fasting here below.

1. For example, if you practice fasting, you may experience bad experiences of irritability, grumpiness, and running toward others. The same can happen when you do intermittent fasting, this is because your body might crave for certain nutrients. If it happens on a regular basis, you should check whether the idea is suitable for you to follow.

2. If you are prone to suffer from depression, intermittent fasting can cause your mood swings to turn into depression. It can also cause anxiety and discouragement. As mentioned earlier, please consult your doctor before starting any diet or intermittent fasting.

3. Most intermittent fasting methods require you to skip breakfast. This can cause brain fog and fatigue. This may not be due to the fact that you are fasting, but it could be because of you are not eating the right foods in your "eating window." Make sure to eat the right food between fasts, and make sure that the food has good fuel for the body.

4. Whenever you restrict your diet through intermittent fasting, you can develop a craving for certain foods. You might develop an obsession with food and can cause psychological problems such as orthorexia. The latter is when you think excessively about food and what you want to eat all day long.

5. One of the major advice here is that you eat a healthy diet. If you do not pay attention to your diet, it will lead to bad eating habits and bad eating habits. In light of the above, you have to think about your meals, but not overthink and obsess over it. Most important of all, you should not binge eat as this issue can lead to a variety of eating disorders (Bradley 2019).

CHAPTER 5: AMONG THE MANY EXAMPLES OF PEOPLE WHO BENEFITED FROM INTERMITTENT FASTING

R ecap the health benefits of intermittent fasting in Chapter 1.

1. The first example here deals with insulin levels, and specifically Type 2 Diabetes. Although it is difficult to prove the research conducted by the Toronto Intensive Diet Management Clinic, it has been shown that intermittent fasting can effectively treat type 2 diabetes.

The clinic conducted an experiment on three patients, and it turned out that their blood sugar levels reached the point where no further insulin treatment was needed. It is clear that intermittently fasting worked for these three diabetics and allowed them to have a significant weight loss as well. However, it must be understood that this was done under strict control (Furmli, Elmasry, Ramos, & Fung). When it comes to medical conditions, in general, treatments such as intermittent fasting should be done under the supervision of your doctor.

2. Intermittent fasting is an excellent way of losing weight. Martine Etienne-Mesubi, who lives in Maryland, Baltimore, USA, weighs 225 pounds, so she actively tries intermittent fasting as a solution. Martine was in a fortunate position that she did research into intermittent fasting

and, therefore, had intimate knowledge of the strategy.

She found that in the past ten years, fasting has become more and more popular, and people have been using it to lose weight, reverse diabetes and even high blood pressure for many years. She started with the experiment and later, it became easier and became a habit in a short time.

She weighed 225 pounds in January 2019 when she started her personal journey, and by April 2019 she had lost 30 pounds. She follows her own way of rule and warns you that you need to follow this weight loss strategy under the guidance of a doctor (Thurrott 2020).

3. The author, James Clear, experimented with intermittent fasting benefited a great deal for him. He found it easier to decide what to eat. It was also a life lesson as he learned to simplify daily decision-making. For example, he does not eat breakfast, and breakfast can easily decide what to eat for lunch, thus simplifying his day.

He found that he had increased energy and reduced body fat. He added that intermittent fasting can even help him make travel plans, especially if healthy food is not available in certain places, as Clear said: During travel, the intermittent fasting schedule can be an important asset (Clear 2019).

4. A personal anecdote might be a good example as well. In general, fasting is as not easy as it deprives the body of one's every day food consumption. Even if you do it for religious purposes, it can be difficult at times. The important thing to note about religious fasting is that you can use intermittent fasting method. Most religions use the 16/8 method, eating one meal in the morning (breakfast) and then eating one meal at around six in the evening.

For certain commemorative events, such as the Muslim holy month of Ramadan, it is usually performed once a year. Christians can, however, fast any time they feel like. They can also choose between any of the intermittent fasting methods discussed at above.

CHAPTER 6: THE
BEST ADVICE FOR
INTERMITTENT FASTING

H ealth is a way to motivate you to try one of the intermittent fasting methods mentioned here. The first step is to make sure you consult your doctor, because your health is the most valuable asset you have (West 2019).

The most important advice for intermittent fasting is the following:

1. Stay Safe

Some of the ways in which to stay safe include:

    i. Consulting your doctor before you start on your intermittent fasting method. It will also serve as a good guide as to which method would be best for you. The more you personalize it the better it will work for you.

    ii. Your choice of fasting method may include eating small portions during the day in order to keep your body stable. This could be a good strategy for you when you start out. Keep the portions small also even after you break your fast.

    iii. Staying hydrated is of paramount importance. Instead of eating something, you can drink fruit juice or dairy products. Here it is important to drink, drinks that are low in calories as well.

2. Know when to stop

As I have said before, it is vital that your doctor has the final say with any of your health choices. However, you should listen to your body, and the moment you feel ill, you should stop your fast. You should also not start fasting when you are unwell. Some things that will suggest that you should stop the fast are:

i.   When you are feeling tired – that is, if you are not able to complete trivial tasks

ii. You should stop immediately if you suddenly feel sick. It is also important to see your doctor if the feeling does not blow over.

iii. If you feel any discomfort, your body is trying to tell you something and you should stop immediately.

3. Stay Focused

Fasting is not always easy, because our nature is to eat.

i.   You can focus on intermittent fasting by taking a walk and focusing on the environment.

ii. You can also meditate in order to keep your mind on the task you set out to do.

iii. You can also do other things, such as art, DIY, or any activity that focuses your attention on hunger.

4. Breaking Your Fast

We know that the warrior method taught us warriors not to eat all day, but to eat a big meal at night. This is just one way describing the method. The idea is that with the fasting methods mentioned here, it is important not to defeat the purpose by overindulging. Therefore, it is best to eat some snacks first, then a small amount of snacks, and then take a break.

5. Watch your Diet

Now you know that intermittent fasting is not a diet, but you should follow the method of choice.

    i.   Intermittent fasting helps cleanse the body. However, if you eat the right food overall, it can help you. This adds to the benefits of, for example, the prevention of cancer, heart diseases, diabetes, and many other chronic diseases.

    ii.   Protein is another valuable food source that will help the body during the fasting. It is especially valuable for building muscle. Most importantly, too, eating small amounts during the day will help control your hunger and appetite.

    iii.   It is vital that you are mindful of what you eat during and after your intermittent fasting.

6. Supplements and Intermittent Fasting

If you are committing to long-term intermittent fasting, your body might begin to miss out on some nutrients. Therefore, it is usually necessary to supplement them. It is best to consult your health practitioner to find out exactly what your body might be missing. It could be anything from potassium to calcium, and most often, the only way to replace it is to use a supplement.

These are just a few things to keep in mind when you want to fast intermittently. You should understand fasting, not for everyone and it requires self-discipline. It is important to have clear reasons and goals for doing this. This will help you keep pace and help you achieve your weight loss goals.

CHAPTER 7: INTERMITTENT FASTING VERSUS OTHER DIETS

A s mentioned earlier, even if intermittent fasting can help you lose weight, it is not a diet in itself. It is a fasting method and is accompanied by a diet, and the diet should be a healthy one. Have a look once more at the different types of intermittent fasting written in Chapter 2. This chapter will focus on the comparison between intermittent fasting and other diets

Intermittent Fasting Versus Calorie Counting

This is a close comparison because it is important to pay attention to calorie intake even if you intermittently fast. *The difference between intermittent fasting and calorie counting is that no matter which type of intermittent fasting method you choose, fasting is the main driver of this strategy.*

> *When using the 5:2 method, men and women are encouraged to limit their calorie intake to 600 and 500 calories, respectively.*

This fact is with every meal after the fast. Even within the fasting regime, it would be inevitable that the calorie intake will be reduced.

However, there is no doubt that calorie counting is a successful diet, but it means a bit more work than when you chose intermittent fasting. With the latter, you will automatically reduce calories, while with a calorie counting diet, you must measure and calculate your daily intake (www.weightlossresources.co.uk).

Intermittent Fasting Versus Intermittent Energy Restriction (Ier) Strategies

Even if you have decided on the type intermittent fasting method, you can still review it and compare with intermittent energy restriction strategies.

The difference is this:

1. Intermittent fasting is the restriction of food for a period of time. This is followed by an extended period of eating where you would eat, for example, within a 4-hour window. As we have noted under "The Warrior Diet," for example, you would not eat for the entire day and then have one big meal at the end of the day.

2. In contrast with intermittent fasting, intermittent energy restriction strategies restrict energy intake to a window of 8-10 hours each day. One big difference is that this is a static way of "fasting" compared to the different ways of intermittent fasting.

3. This also means that you have more leeway in intermittent fasting, because intermittent energy restriction strategies will limit your daily consumption of up to 25% of your energy needs. With intermittent fasting, you can limit your energy intake by 60-100% on the day of the fast and eat as much as possible when the fast is over (Rynders, Corey A et al 2019).

Intermittent Fasting Versus The Ketogenic Diet

1. The Keto diet, which is short for the ketogenic diet, has become as popular as the fasting method. The Keto diet involves control over your carbohydrates. For some people, this means that your daily carbohydrate intake should be less than 50 grams. Others go as low as between 10 and 20 grams. As with any diet, if you restrict your nutritional intake, then if you choose the Keto diet, you need to consult a doctor.

2. With intermittent fasting, you restrict yourself to "eating windows." You have a choice of what you eat within these windows, and can then choose to restrict your carbs or your calories during this time. However, with Keto, you restrict your carbs to less than 50 grams each day. This can lead to nutritional deficiencies.

3. Intermittent fasting gives you more freedom to decide what food to eat, but the keto diet may restrict your diet, and social and psychological difficulties for some people (Munns 2019).

In recent years, the Keto diet has become more mainstream than most of the surrounding diets. It has developed to the point of having specific products ascribed to the diet. It has more so become quite prescriptive as well. As said earlier, intermittent fasting gives you more freedom of choices to choose your foods according to your lifestyle as well.

Intermittent Fasting Versus Traditional Diets

At this point, you already have a sufficient understanding of what intermittent fasting is all about. Even though we are pitting it against the traditional diet, this is exactly the diet you might want to include in your "eating window." This works well because you can eat as many things as you like, and the traditional diet is an excellent guide to healthy eating ("Traditional Diets").

Examples of traditional diets you might want to include in your intermittent fasting regime are:

1. The Mediterranean Diet

The Mediterranean Diet is called this as it covers the traditional foods and means of the people around the Mediterranean Sea. Some of the foods include fruits, vegetables, whole grains, nuts, beans, herbs, spices, and healthy fats. Olive oil is one of the good fats for this diet. It is important to include fish and seafood in your diet at least twice a week. Other foods include fermented dairies such as yogurt and traditional cheese (like feta), eggs, and poultry. Red meat and sweets are rarely eaten and water and wine play a key role.

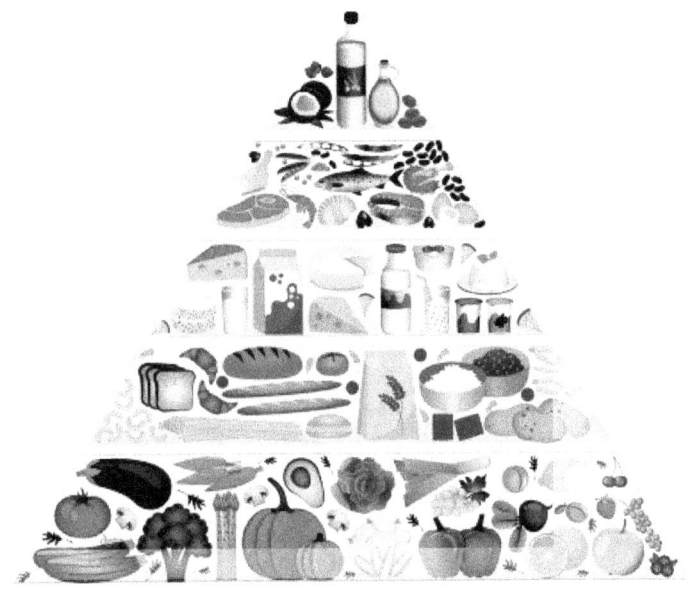

Figure 1: Mediterranean Food Pyramid (free image from Pixabay)

2. The African Heritage Diet

The African Heritage Diet is based on the healthy eating habits of African countries. In addition to being nutritious, these foods are traditionally delicious. Therefore, a meal based on African traditions will be a feast for you. Some of these deliciously healthy foods have their roots in Jamaica and Nigeria. In the USA, the French-Creole foods are fusions of delicious African heritage diets.

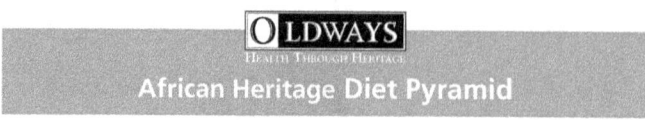

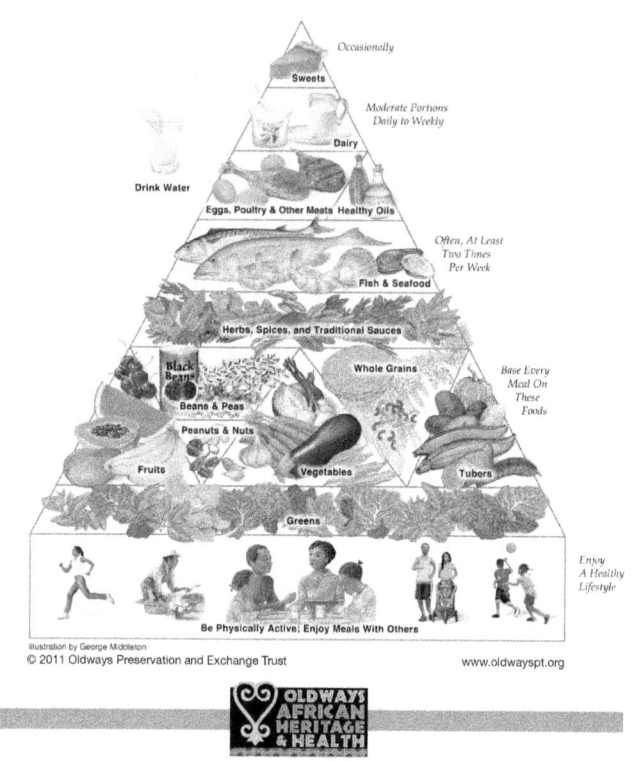

Figure 2: African Heritage Diet Pyramid (https://www.dallasnews.com/news/healthy-living/2018/02/02/free-african-cooking-classes-show-healthy-and-delicious-power-of-heritage/)

3. Latin American Heritage Diet

This diet is based on South American traditions, including Portuguese, Spanish, and large-scale variations of the indigenous peoples of the Mayans, Aztecs, Incas, and many other surrounding countries (called Latin America). The cultures contributed to a pyramid that offers nutrition but also delicious cuisine.

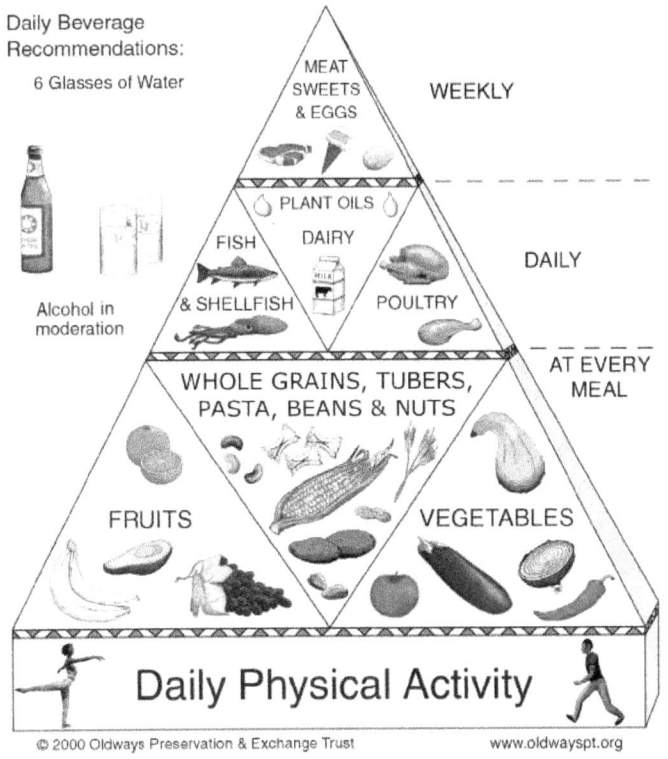

Figure 3: Latin American Food Pyramid (https://www.pinterest.com/pin/497718196295686955/)

The delicious foods mentioned in the pyramids above should serve as motivation for the "eating window" of your intermittent fasting. However, it should also not distract you from your goals.

CHAPTER 8: INTERMITTENT FASTING AND EXERCISE

T he emphasis here would be on safety. It is possible to exercise while you are fasting, but you need to be safe. We repeat, once again, you speak to your doctor about this. When you are chatting with him or her and want to use an intermittent fasting method, exercise should be part of the conversation.

Possible reasons for exercising while on an Intermittent Fasting Regime are as follows:

1. The reason why you might want to exercise while fasting is that you are already on an exercise regime and wish to continue.

2. It is also the fact that you are fasting for religious purposes, and therefore wish to continue your exercise during this time.

3. You are fasting because you want to lose weight and would want to increase the speed of your weight loss.

4. It would also be effective for burning calories

5. Your fasting is important to you as it will increase the shedding of old cells in the body and build new and healthier cells. This is called autophagy.

Exercising during intermittent fasting may have negative results

1. We have noted that reduce your calorie intake during an intermittent fast, and this can affect your muscle-building. This will call for a muscle-building diet within the "eating window."

2. Usually, when you fast, you will find dizziness or light-headedness. This is even more possible when you exercise while you are on your intermittent fasting regime. This may be due to the fact that your blood pressure level may be lower during fasting.

3. Another reason that exercise may have a negative effect is that your blood sugar levels will also drop (as we have already discussed). Exercising while fasting may cause your blood levels to drop so low that you may faint.

We repeat that you should consult your doctor whenever you want to go on a diet, and this includes an intermittent fasting regime. It is even more important that you do so if you combine it with exercise ("Intermittent fasting and exercise: How to do it safely").

CHAPTER 9: INTERMITTENT FASTING AND WEIGHT LOSS

S hould you choose an intermittent fasting regime for weight loss, it is important to consult your doctor. You may be tired of hearing this, but your health is your life and it is therefore extremely important. We have touched on weight loss as part of intermittent fasting, but it is worth looking at how it benefit to you.

The first step to using intermittent fasting to lose weight is to choose which one of the plans you are going to try. You have a choice between the 16:8 method, the 5:2, method, the Warrior Diet, the 'Eat Stop Eat' regime, and the alternate-day fasting (ADF). The methods were discussed in chapter 1.

The second step is to look at how intermittent fasting can help you with your weight loss. There are ways of doing this and here are just a few suggestions.

1. You know that you are overweight, therefore the first thing on the list is to weigh yourself. The reason for this is that you need to keep track of your weight as you progress through the fasting plan.

2. The next aspect is to set up the plan you wish to follow, which is based on the intermittent fasting regime you have chosen.

i. Set up an enlarged chart or calendar on your wall in the kitchen, your study room or bedroom.

ii. Use the online intermittent fasting calculator or the intermittent fasting tracker mobile app to monitor the entire fasting program. It will tell you what you need to eat, calorie calculations, workout split, and all intermittent fasting diet details.

Research has shown that weight loss is possible with intermittent fasting.

The 5:2 method of intermittent fasting can be an effective way to lose weight. This is because not only it can become a weight loss program, but can also become a lifestyle.

Thus, you are able to use it as a continuous weight-watching program as well. Once the weight is off, it is easy to maintain through the 5:2 regime (see chapter 1, Figure 2 for a quick view of this method.

Do remember that, the foods you eat in your "eating window" will have a direct effect on your weight loss as well. Thus, you might want to use this method for a smooth transition into weight loss but more so as a life-long commitment to a healthy body.

The 16:8 intermittent fasting method is an easy way of losing weight. This is because it allows you to drink low-calorie beverages during a 16-hour period.

A few studies dispute the fact that one can lose weight with this type of fasting. It seems almost like a normal day for most working people (Trepanowski et al). Most workers often skip breakfast, just drink water, and other beverages throughout the day, then eat their first meal at lunchtime.

They would then eat their last meal at eight in the evening because they need to have an early night for work the next day. Therefore, if you work together to eat the right food during the 8 to 10 hour feeding period, this method may only be effective for weight loss. There are health benefits, and even though there are disputes, the diet you follow with this method will determine whether you lose weight or not.

The previous chapters mentioned the reduction of calories could be an important aspect of weight loss. In light of this, intermittent fasting increases your metabolism, which is directly responsible for burning calories. This inevitably leads to weight loss.

> As discussed in chapter 2, intermittent fasting has an effect on belly fat as well. Losing belly fat is an important reason why most people would choose this type of fasting as it would increase your metabolism by 3.6-14% and, thus, help you burn more calories (Gunnars 2016).

> As mentioned before as well, intermittent fasting helps reduce calories and, hence, resulted in weight loss (Barnosky, Hoddy, Unterman, & Varady 2014)

Weight loss is definitely one of the health benefits of intermittent fasting. However, the best option to lose weight would be the Alternate-day fasting method as it is an easier way of doing it. The body can adapt to it more easily, and quicker than with any of the other regimes.

The reason for this is that you would be fast on alternative days for 24 hours each week. However, you have the option of eating limited calories instead of fasting on those alternative days. See Figure 4 for a quick view of the program (Clayton

2019). This fact is effective for a quick weight loss program as it is also psychologically easier.

According to the research of researchers Welton et al., 27 subjects who fasted on alternate-days lost 0.8% to 13.0% of their baseline body weight within 12 weeks.

They also determined that most of the weight loss caused by intermittent fasting is fat loss. We have looked at this in the calorie-burning aspect in chapter 3 with how the liver deals with this matter.

They concluded that the study indicated that there is promise in the treatment of obesity in particular. However, as mentioned throughout the booklet, the consensus is that it can be effective for normal weight loss (Welton, Stephanie et al, 2020).

CONCLUSION

The hope is that this booklet has given you a reasonable overview of what the intermittent fasting regime is about. This book tries to provide you with information and some guidelines about this different type of diet. We have determined that it is not a diet, but a diet that involves fasting.

Some of the aspects we discussed here included:
- The different types of intermittent fasting

- The pros and cons of intermittent fasting

- The health benefits you could get from it

- What side effects you might expect and a few solutions for these side effects

- We provide some examples of people who have benefited from intermittent fasting, that included personal experiences of the fasting regime.

- The advice we provided is a general overview of what you might expect from intermittent fasting and what to do when you fast.

- We have also looked at how intermittent fasting compares to other diets, particularly Calorie Counting, Intermittent Energy Restriction (IER) Strategies, the Ketogenic Diet, and Traditional Diets.

There is a wealth of information about intermittent fasting, and the information here is just the tip of the iceberg. You are free to choose which plan you want to follow, and it is important that you use this as the foundation for your own research. You choose for what purpose you want to fast – that includes fasting for religious purposes or for weight loss.

Most importantly, the booklet also showed you the health benefits as well as the negative aspects of intermittent fasting. It is safe to say that the benefits outweigh the negatives. Also, you need to be sure that you consult your doctor especially if you are going to exercise while fasting as well. We have also determined that intermittent fasting is good for health and helps to lose weight.

An important aspect throughout the process is that it is possible to use any intermittent fasting method to improve your health, but if this is your goal, you can also lose weight

References

Barnosky, Adrienne R., et al. "Intermittent Fasting vs Daily Calorie Restriction for Type
2 Diabetes Prevention: a Review of Human Findings." *Translational Research*, vol. 164, no. 4, 2014, pp. 302–311., doi:10.1016/j.trsl.2014.05.013.

Bradley, Sarah. "If You Have Any Of These Intermittent Fasting Side Effects, It Might
Mean IF Isn't A Great Fit For You." *Women's Health*, 12 Nov. 2019, www.womenshealthmag.com/weight-loss/a29657614/intermittent-fasting-side-effects/.

Clayton, David. "Intermittent Fasting: What's the Best Method?" *Medical Xpress –*
Medical Research Advances and Health News, Medical Xpress, 7 June 2019, medicalxpress.com/news/2019-06-intermittent-fasting-method.html#:~:text=While 5:2 could be,a very low calorie diet.

Clear, James. "The Good and The Bad of Intermittent Fasting: 2 Years of
Experiments." *James Clear*, 4 Feb. 2019, jamesclear.com/good-bad-intermittent-fasting.

Goodrick, C. L., et al. "Differential Effects of Intermittent Feeding and Voluntary
Exercise on Body Weight and Lifespan in Adult Rats." *Journal of Gerontology*, vol. 38, no. 1, 1983, pp. 36–45., doi:10.1093/geronj/38.1.36.

Gunnars, Kris. "10 Evidence-Based Health Benefits of Intermittent Fasting." *Healthline*,
Healthline Media, 16 Aug. 2016, www.healthline.com/nutrition/10-health-benefits-of-intermittent-fasting#TOC_TITLE_HDR_2.

_ _. "What Is Intermittent Fasting? Explained in Human Terms." *Healthline*,
Healthline Media, 4 June 2017, www.healthline.com/nutrition/what-is-intermittent-fasting#TOC_TITLE_HDR_2.

_ _. "6 Popular Ways to Do Intermittent Fasting." *Healthline*, Healthline
Media, 2 Jan. 2020, www.healthline.com/nutrition/6-ways-to-do-intermittent-fasting#TOC_TITLE_HDR_4.

Harvard Health. "Not so Fast: Pros and Cons of the Newest Diet
Trend." *Harvard Health Publishing*, www.health.harvard.edu/heart-health/not-so-fast-pros-and-cons-of-the-newest-diet-trend.

"Intermittent Fasting and Exercise: How to Do It Safely." *Medical News Today*,
MediLexicon International, www.medicalnewstoday.com/articles/intermittent-fasting-and-working-out#why-it-might-not.

Kubala, Jillian. "The Warrior Diet: Review and Beginner's Guide." *Healthline*,
Healthline Media, 3 July 2018, www.healthline.com/nutrition/warrior-diet-guide.

Lawler, Moira, et al. "12 Possible Intermittent Fasting Benefits: Everyday
Health." *EverydayHealth.com*, www.everydayhealth.com/diet-nutrition/possible-intermittent-fasting-benefits/.

Munns, Diane. "Intermittent Fasting vs Keto: Which Is Better for Weight
Loss?" *Bodyandsoulau*, Bodyandsoul.com.au, 3 Mar. 2019, www.bodyandsoul.com.au/diet/lose-weight/intermittent-fasting-vs-keto-whats-better-for-weight-loss/news-story/744c69595dd7af5fb00752627ad4cdc8.

Owings, Justin."Getting Started With 16:8 Intermittent Fasting on The Leangains Method
Diet." *Justin Owings*, justinowings.com/getting-started-with-168-intermittent-fasting-on-the-leangains-method-diet/.

Rynders, Corey A et al. "Effectiveness of Intermittent Fasting and Time-Restricted
Feeding Compared to Continuous Energy Restriction for Weight Loss." *Nutrients* vol. 11,10 2442. 14 Oct. 2019, doi:10.3390/nu11102442

The Mayo Clinic Staff. "Diabetes Treatment: Using Insulin to Manage Blood
Sugar." *Mayo Clinic*, Mayo Foundation for Medical Education and Research, 24 July 2019, www.mayoclinic.org/diseases-conditions/diabetes/in-depth/diabetes-treatment/art-20044084.

Thompson, Dennis. "'Intermittent Fasting' Diet Could Boost Your Health." *WebMD*,
WebMD, 26 Dec. 2019, www.webmd.com/diet/news/20191226/intermittent-fasting-diet-could-boost-your-health#1.

Thurrott, Stephanie. "How One Woman Used Intermittent Fasting to Lose 80 Pounds in a
Year." *NBCNews.com*, NBCUniversal News Group, 28 Jan. 2020, www.nbcnews.com/better/lifestyle/how-one-woman-used-intermittent-fasting-lose-80-pounds-year-ncna1124121.

"Traditional Diets." *Oldways*, oldwayspt.org/traditional-diets.

Trepanowski JF, Kroeger CM, Barnosky A, Klempel MC, Bhutani S, Hoddy KK, Gabel
K, Freels S, Rigdon J, Rood J, Ravussin E, Varady

KA. Effect of Alternate-Day Fasting on Weight Loss, Weight Maintenance, and Cardioprotection Among Metabolically Healthy Obese Adults: A Randomized Clinical Trial. JAMA Intern Med. 2017 Jul 1;177(7):930-938. doi: 10.1001/jamainternmed.2017.0936. PMID: 28459931; PMCID: PMC5680777.

Welton, Stephanie et al. "Intermittent fasting and weight loss: Systematic
    review." *Canadian family physician Medecin de famille canadien* vol. 66,2 (2020): 117-125.

West, Helen. "How to Fast Safely: 10 Helpful Tips." *Healthline*, Healthline Media, 2 Jan.
    2019,   www.healthline.com/nutrition/how-to-fast#TOC_TITLE_HDR_5.

Www.weightlossresources.co.uk. "Intermittent Fasting VS Calorie Counting - Actually It
    Doesn't Matter." *Weight Loss Resources*, www.weightlossresources.co.uk/news/any-diet-just-do-it.htm.

AFTERWORD

Did You Like This Book?

Please consider leaving a positive review and give me 4 to 5 stars on the customer review page?

Even just a few positive words would help others to decide if the book is right for them. And it is much appreciate.

Contact Me.

Email: eclickzonetrading@gmail.com

Thank you.

www.ingramcontent.com/pod-product-compliance
Lightning Source LLC
Chambersburg PA
CBHW071115220526
45467CB00004B/1896